I0765844

The Quick Start Guide to Autophagy for Beginners

The Quick Start Guide to Autophagy for Beginners

–

Discover how to activate autophagy for weight loss, good health, and longevity.

GWENDOLYN MYERS

Table of Contents

Introduction

◆ ◆ ◆

Let's start this book with a series of questions. What if there was an easy way to remove all the harmful substances from your body? What if there was an amazing recycling system within your body that can clean up everything that has been stored for years? What if there was a way to live longer? What if there was an easy way to lose weight? So many questions, right? Here, in this book, you will find all the answers. Just keep reading...

A friend of mine wanted to lose weight so badly that she had tried so many diets and exercise regimes and none of them were of much help. I guess many of you have had the same problem. She had so many other health problems all due to her being overweight. Doctors advised her to lose weight, and she did try almost every method she had heard of, but it did not end up with success. She would lose weight, but after some time, it just came back. And it was the most discouraging feeling she had ever felt in her life. She tried over and over again, but the results were always the same. These rigorous diets were just giving her some instant results, but since they weren't meant to be part of a lifestyle, the weight just kept coming back.

Finally, with my help, she found out about autophagy and I explained to her how this amazing process works. She started changing her lifestyle one step at a time and by doing that, she not only lost weight, but also burned fat and did so many positive things to her overall health that everyone was just simply amazed. Of course, the happiest of them all was my friend because she achieved her goal fairly easy and she had never felt better in her life. The reason behind this is the fact that autophagy does not only help you to lose weight, but it has numerous other health benefits. I love to think of it as a fountain of health and youth. This breathtaking process will clear out your body from the inside and this is what matters. You know those apples and peaches that start rotting from the middle. When you look at them from the outside they look great, delicious and healthy, but when you cut them open, you realize that they are rotten inside and barely anything is edible. Now, the same goes for humans. Well, not identical, no one is going to eat humans, but you get the idea. There are tiniest pieces of humans that cannot be seen with naked eye and within those elements, there are buildups of so many negative and harmful components that if you do not clean them up, they can grow to become a very difficult illness. However, there are innate body systems that are made for such jobs and they do clean up the body. But what if those processes have some kind of a glitch and are not working properly? We need to help our bodies with the methods that are presented here, in this book, in order to cleanse from within.

This book is divided into three major parts. Two of these parts cover the basics of autophagy, what it is and how it works. Also, you are given instructions on what you can do to help your body induce autophagy. These two parts cover numerous researches and the results of these studies which only prove and give you a better perspective of how important this process is for our health and wellbeing. Through my research and some personal insights, I was amazed by the strong relationship between autophagy and inducing this process regularly and the overall health of a person. Inducing the process of autophagy not only helps you burn fat, but it also helps your body recycle and regenerate at lower levels.

You will also see how autophagy is used to prevent and treat different diseases and disorders. There are many scientific researches and proofs that autophagy or the lack of it can be one of the reasons some diseases and disorders appear. Therefore, this process is not being researched for all its benefits and possibilities of how different diseases can be treated using regulation of the autophagy process. There are some very interesting studies yet to be conducted, so this field of study is going to give us even more information about the processes that are going on inside our bodies in the future.

The third part of this book is focused mostly on different diets and exercise that will help you induce the process of autophagy. Of course, before starting any of these methods, you should first consult your physician.

This book contains proven steps and strategies on how to induce autophagy and help your own body get regenerated. You will benefit from autophagy induction in many ways. As you will find out from the chapters of this book, autophagy is the key process that is important for normal functioning of the body. I hope that this book will inspire you to take care of your health even more, regardless of whether you need to lose weight or not. It is possible to live a long and healthy life with just a little help from the inside.

Let's learn how!

Chapter One: What is Autophagy?

◆ ◆ ◆

Imagine you live in a house that never gets cleaned. Imagine a street that has no garbage bins. Imagine a planet filled with garbage. Now, imagine a body that keeps its waste and doesn't discharge it. Oh, wait. That is not the right way to look at things. We do clean after ourselves and we do care about our planet. So, why don't we take care of our bodies too?

If only we did something to clean our bodies as easily. Well, there is a way. Autophagy is a process that helps our bodies get rid of all the bad things that are collected over the time. The word autophagy itself has a very disturbing meaning. It comes from Greek words *auto*, which means self, and *phagy*, which means self. Therefore, the literal meaning of the word autophagy is self-eating or self-devouring. It is really almost impossible to imagine that our bodies are capable of eating themselves up. However, studies have proven that there is a process that occurs inside each living being that actually resembles this self-devouring idea. The process itself may not visible, but the results definitely are. In fact, there are many proofs that cells within our bodies are cannibals. They are able to eat parts of them that are damaged or misplaced or generally harmful for the rest of the organism.

From the scientific point of view, autophagy is a natural mechanism that regulates and retains beneficial substances while it removes all the harmful substances from the body. It is, in fact, 'playing a housekeeping role in the elimination of misfolded or aggregated proteins, the eradication of damaged organelles, proteins, and cancerous materials, and the elimination of foreign pathogens such as viruses via a degrading lysosomal pathway.' (Khandia et al., 2019) This means that autophagy is responsible for taking care and protecting the good parts of cells as well as for the removal of all the negative and harmful cell parts. It reduces the negative processes that can occur in the body system and helps you regenerate.

To better understand this, think of the human body as a recycling system. Within each human body, there are good and beneficial substances, as well as those that are harmful. Your body is trained to go through all the harmful substances and eliminate and destroy them while still using the outcome of this self-eating process to produce energy or to build new cells. This way, you not only get the benefits of removing the cellular waste, but you also gain through energy and new cells building. This is the essence of the process in which components inside the cells are destroyed, degraded and recycled. This process is called autophagy and it is a natural way to regulate the amounts of beneficial and harmful substances inside the body.

However, this does not happen by itself. It actually can happen by itself and it does occur normally from time to time, but since the life has nowadays become so busy and we don't have time to think about what and how and when we eat, we may unintentionally stop our bodies from activating autophagy. In order to trigger autophagy, one has to get their body in a state of stress. This does not include the psychological stress we all go through from time to time. This means that the body needs to go through food deprivation or through intense body workout in order to kick-start autophagy. The body needs to feel threatened by some sort of stress in order to begin regenerating and renewing on a cellular level. This happens if you exercise or have an intense body activity or are exposed to some sort of starvation. When you are exercising your muscles are actually experiencing tiny, micro fractures and lacerations that your body is trying to repair as quickly as possible. This is the reason why you may feel sore after a workout. On a cellular level, your cells are actually removing all the malfunctioning and harmful parts and renewing and producing the good cells. In other words, the process of autophagy begins. Another way of kick-starting autophagy is fasting. You can either fast for certain foods or you can fast entirely from all foods and get your body to start the process of autophagy on cellular level. If you think you cannot endure a 12-hour or even longer fasts which rule out all types of food, then, there are other solutions. You can try one of the well thought out diets that exclude the intake of carbohydrates and sugars. You will see later on that the reduction of carbohydrates and sugars is crucial when it comes to autophagy. The best way to kick-start autophagy is to fast intermittently. If you are not familiar with intermittent fasting, it is simply fasting throughout 12, 24, 36, 48 or more hours. During that time, you can choose to either avoid all foods and drinks or you can just have good, old plain water to keep your body hydrated. Water is also the most ideal and the healthiest liquid to maintain your body hydration. If you are planning to fast for longer periods of time, you will need to consult your physician to make sure you won't have further health complications due to longer fasting periods.

When your body is well fed, the cells are in a state of growth. To put it simply, they have plenty of nutrients to grow from and they don't bother about recycling and all that. The mTOR (i.e. mammalian target of rapamycin) pathways that direct the cells to grow, divide themselves and synthesize proteins are highly active in that state. Such cells, which are well-fed, do not care about recycling and reorganizing the structures, but they are focused on growing and dividing. This may seem as a good thing, but in fact, it is not. If the cells continue growing and dividing, without cleaning up the waste, your organism may get into a bad state, which may result in metabolic or neurodegenerative diseases, for example. Therefore, it is important that everyone tries to fast at least once a month to clean their bodies from all the toxins that are accumulated over the time.

When it comes to intermittent fasting, there are several stages that your body goes through. These don't have to be identical for everyone, but they are more or less the same. After you have fasted for 12 hours, your body starts burning fat and it enters into a metabolic state that is known as ketosis. This is a state where your body breaks down and burns the fat from your body and then, this fat is used by your liver to produce ketones or ketone bodies. These will serve as an alternative source of energy for your brain cells and for the cells in other tissues once your body gets into this state and glucose and other sugars aren't readily available.

Several hours later, your body will produce much higher levels of ketones that will be used to fuel your brain and other organs. The usage of ketones by your brain is better than glucose because it is less inflammatory, and it can boost your memory. This is also why fasting is so closely connected to positive mood and mental clarity. Autophagy starts to take place within 24 hours of fasting and there is significant change on a cellular level. Your cells are starting to recycle some of their components, and they are repurposing them. The recycled 'material' is used as an energy fuel or as new components for new cells.

By the time you are fasting for 48 hours, with little to no calorie intake, your hormone of growth is increased by four to five times when compared to its level when you just started fasting. Ketones, combined with hunger hormone, ghrelin, both force the body to produce more growth hormones.

These hormones in change provide the preservation of lean muscle mass and the reduction of accumulation of fat tissues in the body. In the next stages, your body will experience low insulin levels, which will cause insulin sensitivity, and after 72 hours of fasting, your body will start to break down the old immune cells and it will start generating new ones. This insulin sensitivity may be very good for your overall health, since it may bring many benefits, such as lowering the chances of developing diabetes as well as of some other chronic diseases that come with age. The more you keep yourself away from the carbohydrates and sugars, the better. Your body will be forced to use up the fats that have been stored in your body and this will, in turn, generate ketones that will become the fuel for your brain and other organs. The most important thing is that not only will you get healthier; you may also lose weight during the process. However, with fasting, you do not lose muscle mass, but only fats, which is the best and the healthiest way to lose weight. But once you are finished with fasting, there is one more stage to this process and that is refeeding. You will, naturally, need to start eating regularly, again. You should start refeeding gradually, without taking large amounts of food at once, but start with smaller meals and take breaks between eating, so you're your body has time to adapt to new situation. What you will want to avoid is, same as you did during the fasting period, carbohydrates and sugars. These are difficult to process, and your cells will again start growing and duplicating. Consuming lots of sugars and carbohydrates might also lead to problems with blood sugar, since your organism was led to a stage where it became insulin sensitive. Therefore, you don't want to exaggerate with anything. You should finish your fast with a balanced meal that has plenty of vegetables that contain fibers and fats, as well as some healthy proteins. You can also add a portion of whole wheat cereals. The important thing is that you choose what suits you the best, but be careful not to go overboard with sugar.

So, as you could see and notice yourself, our bodies do contain its very own recycling system. Our body is capable of recycling all the malfunctioning parts to create more energy or to create new, functioning cells. It is one amazing system. If you look at it from a different perspective, you will notice that these situations we can go through are quite dangerous. If there were no mechanism like this one, situations like starvation and highly intense exercise might actually kill us. I know that in many cases it really does lead to one's death. However, human body is adapting to these stressful situations by taking advantage of the state they're in. Instead of collapsing, something amazing happens on a cellular level. Autophagy kicks in and cells experience a recycling cycle. They go from a state they've been in to a completely cleaned out and reorganized state. On a cellular level, bad and harmful components of cells are ruled out and they are either transformed into energy or they are used as material for the formation of new cells.

Chapter Two: Scientific Background

◆ ◆ ◆

From a scientific point of view, autophagy is a very important process that occurs within our bodies. It may be a crucial element in maintaining one's health. It is a 'physiological cellular process through which intracellular components undergo lysosome-mediated self-digestion and recycling.' (Netea-Maier, Plantinga, van de Veerdonk, Smit, & Netea, 2015) Autophagy has a vital role in the maintenance of cellular homeostasis and through that role it is involved in modulating cell metabolism, host defense and survival of cells. In other words, it maintains stability within the cells while it is adjusting to the conditions that are new to the cells. That is exactly what homeostasis is; on a cellular level, it is a cell self-regulating system which enables cells to maintain stability.

Conditions such as hypoxia, exposure to some toxic molecule or starvation can trigger autophagy to get activated and all of that is happening so that the cellular stability is maintained. The number of researches that confirm and support the idea of involvement of autophagy in numerous physiological processes, such as cell survival, cell metabolism, host defense and others, has emerged recently. Some researches argue that autophagy might the earliest form of innate immunity of eukaryotes against microorganisms that are invading them. However, researches also argue that mammals have evolved these primeval autophagy functions and now have many adaptive and innate mechanisms of immunity. Furthermore, defective autophagy recently gets more and more connected to several pathological diseases or conditions, like neurodegenerative disease, autoimmune disease, senescence and cancer.

These newer researches show that autophagy besides being a good 'housekeeper' of one's body; it is the most crucial element in host defending, and in regulating the inflammations that occur in a body. The research has shown that autophagy does improve the host defense mechanisms and it does so through several biological functions, and these are: directly eliminating the pathogens that are invading a body system, controlling adaptive immunity by regulating how antigen are handled and presented, inducing innate or trained immunity memory and modulating inflammations. Having all this presented, one can indeed come to a conclusion that autophagy is 'an ancient form of innate immune response to an infection.' (Netea-Maier, et al., 2015)

So, in the core of the matter, we have a cellular process which recycles proteins that are long-lived, as well as some damaged organelles, and in that process it maintains energy stability. These organelles and proteins are then separated into a double-membrane structure which is called autophagosome, which then connects with lysosomes in order to degrade the malfunctioning and harmful components. Even though it is originally classified as one of the types of cell deaths that are programmed, nowadays, it is more viewed as a basic mechanism of cell survival that actually fights against environmental stressors. These genes were primarily found and identified in yeast and through examining, conclusion that autophagy genes are necessary to avoid starvation and stress caused by lack of nutrients. Once these genes were noticed in mammals, their mammalian counterparts only confirmed how important they are for a normal development of an organism.

What happens inside a cell is amazing. As I said earlier, one cannot see the process, well, not everyone can see it. Scientists have proven that autophagosomes are formed inside the cells. Autophagy occurs in several stages and it results in mature autophagosomes. First stage is de novo forming a double-membrane structure which is also called phagophore. The second stage is elongating this membrane that is lipid-based. And the third and final stage is encapsulating the intracellular cargo from which a mature autophagosome will be formed. These autophagosomes fuse with lysosomes and form autolysosomes, which then proceed to degrading and recycling the components so that it may maintain the energy stability inside the cell.

Now, the situations that trigger these processes are various, as you could see. They vary from starvation to some other, more physical stressors. However, the most widely used autophagy inhibitor is starvation. Starvation-induced autophagy facilitates the degradation of lipids, carbohydrates and proteins, which helps cells to adapt to new conditions and therefore, cells can maintain energy homeostasis. The research has shown that when it comes to newborn mice, autophagy plays the most important role once the supply with nutrients that occurred via placenta ends. It seemed that thanks to autophagy, various tissues of these newborn mice were able to maintain certain energy levels, even after the nutrient supplies ceased. Furthermore, this type of autophagy, the starvation-induced, blocks the mitochondria to induce the apoptosis and as a result, we can say that it has cytoprotective effect to a cell.

However, if the autophagy is not regulated, it may cause some disorders, such as infectious and metabolic diseases, neurodegenerative disorders and cancer. In some cases, it may happen that autophagy is prevented, and this may happen in any stage of the process and it may cause the progression of disease. On the other hand, there has been evidence that autophagy can increase longevity in many species, which raises the possibility that autophagy induction can be used even for ageing and longevity purposes. Given that one may be able to control the process of autophagy, we may only imagine that regulating it may benefit patients with neurodegenerative diseases, while there would be possible to prevent autophagy in treating some cancers, as some researches indicate.

All in all, autophagy is an important process that occurs within our bodies on a cellular level. It most definitely helps us to live healthier and possibly longer. The key for health is yet to be found, but it is close to autophagy.

Chapter Three: Autophagy in Cancer Treatments

◆ ◆ ◆

When it comes to cancer treatments and involvement of autophagy in it, it may get complicated. It is the first disorder that was connected to lack of autophagy, and it is also the first disorder whose treatments were actually inhibiting autophagy. It may seem confusing, but once you get into it, it makes sense. One of the reasons why cancer cells even begin growing is the lack of autophagy within the body, so much so that these cells begin growing and dividing, sometimes at an astonishing pace. However, when it comes to treating the illness, it is inhibited in order not to work on these harmful cells and give them even more power and energy. 'The prevailing current view is that autophagy functions both as a tumor suppressor pathway that prevents tumor initiation and as a pro-survival pathway that helps tumor cells endure metabolic stress and resist death triggered by chemotherapeutic agents.' (Rubinsztein, Codogno, & Levine, 2012)

Even though there is great complexity in what causes tumor to progress and if autophagy has a great role in that process, there is still general consensus and that is the fact that autophagy itself does suppress the initiation of tumors. 'Genetic deletion of the autophagy gene BECN1 is associated with enhanced susceptibility to breast, ovarian and prostate cancer in humans and increased spontaneous malignancies in mice. Mice deficient in ATG4C show increased susceptibility to chemically-induced fibrosarcomas, and mice with deletion of Atg5 or Atg7 develop benign liver tumors.' (Rubinsztein, et al., 2012) As we can see, there is a lot of evidence that certain gene mutations may promote tumorigenesis, as well as how a lack of autophagy can lead to such mutations.

Moreover, autophagy does regulate the properties of stem-cells of cancer by 'contributing to the maintenance of stemness, the induction of recurrence, and the development of resistance to anticancer reagents.' It is clear that one has to be very careful in treating diseases like cancer. There are some autophagy modulators that are used in regulating autophagy in therapy against cancer, like rapamycin and chloroquine. However, these are used to regulate between suppression and promotion of tumor and even though there have been practices of regulating autophagy, it still needs a lot of research before one can say that they have a cure for cancer.

Research has shown that when it comes to cancer biology, there are two roles that autophagy may have and these are of tumor promoting and tumor suppressing, while it can contribute to cancer cells to develop and proliferate. Some drugs that are used against cancer can actually regulate autophagy. Thus, chemotherapy that regulates autophagy can lead to the survival or removal of cancer cells. Furthermore, autophagy regulation can contribute to 'the tumor suppressor proteins or oncogenes. Tumor suppressor factors are negatively regulated by mTOR and AMPK, resulting in the induction of autophagy and suppression of the cancer initiation. In contrast, oncogenes may be activated by mTOR, class I PI3K, and AKT, resulting in the suppression of autophagy and enhancement of cancer formation.' (Yun & Lee, 2018) This means that if one is able to control whether autophagy can be activated at a certain time, and not oncogenes, they might be able to prevent the formation of cancer cells.

If autophagy is reduced or abnormal, it can inhibit degradation of proteins or damaged components of cells into oxidative stressed cells, which then lead to cancer development. As you could see, autophagy can be considered to be one of factors of suppressing cancer and cancer prevention. Research has shown that if some important autophagy proteins mutate, they can suppress tumor development. For example, 'BIF-1 proteins that are related to BECN1 have been observed to become abnormal or absent in variety of cancer types, such as colorectal and gastric cancer.' (Yun & Lee, 2018) There is also evidence that UVRAG proteins are related to BECN1, and that they can also regulate autophagy. If UVRAG proteins mutate, they will reduce autophagy, which will result in an increase of cancer cells proliferating in colorectal cancer. However, when it comes to some other types of cancer, like RAS-activated one, such as pancreatic one, there is high level of basal autophagy. When increased autophagy is constrained, in such cancers there is a decrease in cancer cell proliferation and a suppression of cancer occurs. Thus, one can claim that autophagy does have a crucial role in both initiating and suppressing of tumors and tumor development.

In my humble opinion, autophagy can be used as prevention for such illnesses, because if you trigger autophagy at least once or twice a month, there is less chance that all those harmful cellular components will build up. You will clean up your body and as a result, you may rest assured that it is less likely that any tumorous cells that may threaten your health will be formed. Additionally, if you do find yourself in such state and condition, you should stay positive and do what is in your ability to overcome such disease. As far as the research goes, this field is in its beginning phases of researching. There are many causes and effects that need yet to be discovered. All things considered, one may hope that in future, cancer will become a thing of past and that one will be able to prevent and to reduce and annihilate cancer cells by regulating their inner processes, primarily autophagy.

Chapter Four: Autophagy as a Key Factor in Cell Regeneration

◆ ◆ ◆

As it was already mentioned a couple of times, autophagy is the key process in maintaining stability (homeostasis) within cells. While cells are under normal conditions, they use basal autophagy levels to help maintain biological function, stability, control the quality of the cell contents and they eliminate long-lived proteins and organelles that are damaged. Furthermore, when it comes to stem cells, autophagy is related to maintaining the unique properties of stem cells, which includes self-renewal and differentiation.

Satellite cells, which are actually stem cells of skeletal muscles, are the ones who are responsible for the ability of skeletal muscles to regenerate. These satellite cells are usually found in a state of resting, which is called quiescence. They are activated once damage is made to the muscle tissue. In tissues that are like skeletal muscles, the state of quiescence that is reversible is the regular, normal state which stays the same in one's lifetime. However, there are some recent studies that show that this normal state of resting of these stem cells is changed at geriatric stage of life to an irreversible senescence state, which, in turn, will result in a decrease of quantity and function of these cells and most probably in a failure of possibility for muscles to regenerate.

Recent studies show that autophagy plays a key role in maintaining stem cells at their best. One such study that was carried out 'on mice of different ages demonstrates that satellite cells in young mice are equipped with protecting quality control mechanisms, such as autophagy, that actively repress the senescence program, thus preserving cell integrity and aptitude.' (Garcia-Prat, et al., 2018) The research has proven that when autophagy process fails, it will cause aging to start and it will result in accumulating misfolded proteins and damaged organelles within stem cells and that will lead to exhaustion and senescence. As a demonstration, researchers went on to genetically inhibit autophagy within satellite cells of young mice and that caused satellite cells to enter into state of senescence and this state soon resulted in failure of muscle regeneration.

This research also proved how restoring autophagy reversed senescence and how it restored functions that are related to regeneration of those long-lived satellite cells. The research also revealed that the restoration of autophagy is the key element in the regulating eradication of the stem cells, and as such, it has the potential to be the most important strategy in fighting against the inability of muscle regeneration in conditions like sarcopenia, which is a state of losing muscle mass which is caused by inactivity and ageing.

Pura Muñoz-Cánoves, who is the leading researcher in this study claims that with this research, they have identified autophagy, or more importantly failing to induce this process, is the 'determining factor of the regenerative capacity in muscle stem cells in the aged.' (Garcia-Prat, et al., 2018) She also claims that this research will lead to investigating 'the loss of regenerative capacity of the muscle in elderly people' and therefore, we will be able to help elderly address the issues they have and give them better life quality in overall.

There are numerous experiments that were conducted in order to come to conclusions as to what helps cells to regenerate. One such experiment is conducted on zebrafish. In this experiment, researchers surgically amputated the caudal fin of the zebrafish. What followed this amputation is the formation of blastema by dedifferentiation of cells that were nearest to the cut. This blastema then re-differentiated in order to regenerate the part of the fin that was amputated. What is interesting is that cell types do not change, and they remain stable during the process. Also, there was a noticeable increase in the expression of protein ATG8 in cells that are nearest to the cut, as well as later on in blastema. The number of the autophagosomes was also visibly increased.

Given that many, if not all of the experiments were conducted on animals, there might be some connection to what happens in human body. Of course, this does not mean that these processes are identical to what happens to humans, but when observing what occurs in the cells and molecules of animals, in particular mammals, one may come to conclusions that similar processes may occur in human body as well. The bottom line is that autophagy and its proper functioning is the key element in cellular regeneration and that if one could control autophagy, they might be able to regenerate some parts on purpose, so to say.

This, in fact, means that if one has issues on a cellular level, autophagy is the system that may help them restore and re-establish stability. As we could see, autophagy is crucial in maintaining cellular homeostasis or stability and through this process, it not only cleans, but also regenerates cells and through all those processes we remain healthy.

Chapter Five: Role of Autophagy in Toxin Removal

♦♦♦

If we put it in a simple and easy to understand words, autophagy is the recycling system of our bodies. By now, you have figured that it happens on a cellular level and through this process, cells remain in their balanced out state. However, over time, even though body removes toxin regularly, there are those tiny bits and pieces that still remain and build up over time. This is where autophagy comes into place. It not only helps cells remain in homeostasis, but it helps cells clean up. This process helps our bodies to remove all the misfolded proteins, damaged organelles and other harmful components. This is done on a cellular level in several stages where cells form a membrane which increases and gathers all of the negative components that need to be removed and together with lysosome they work on degrading these components and creating energy for cells or they will be used as a basis for new cells. This is best observed in intermittent fasting, where the cells don't have the carbohydrates and sugars that they would naturally feed on, so they turn to burning down all the nutrients they could get, and this turns out to be the most beneficial process that helps you get and most probably stay healthy.

As you could see from the previous examples and researches, autophagy plays a great role in toxin removal. It not only helps your body to remove all the harmful and negative components within the body, but by doing this clean-up, you will most probably protect your body from many conditions and diseases that are very harmful and invasive for your entire organism. This toxin removal can be beneficial in preventing cancer, as we discussed earlier, as well as in some neurodegenerative and metabolic diseases.

According to many researches, autophagy is of utmost importance for the neuronal homeostasis. If the autophagy is not regulated in the right manner, it may cause numerous neurodegenerative conditions. Due to accumulation of toxic and damaged molecules, one may end up having pathological consequences that manifest themselves in neurodegenerative diseases, such as

Parkinson's, Huntington's and Alzheimer's diseases. Same thing happens if some other toxic waste collects within cells. They may proliferate into cancer cells and, again, we may find ourselves in a fight against a disease that may have serious consequences to our lives. Another very similar outcome may happen and that is problem with metabolic disorders. Due to unhealthy lifestyle, lack of exercise, and plenty of unhealthy food, one may end up having many metabolic problems, and they may end up having lots of excess weight, as well as some other conditions that follow these disorders. However, practicing intermittent fasting from time to time may give you the benefits of preventing or even fixing and repairing some of the damage you did to your body. Regardless of whether these disorders and diseases are genetically transmitted or whether they are result of bad habits and environmental circumstances, one may do their best and induce autophagy to make sure that their body is clean of toxins and that cells are in their optimal state. Be sure that whenever you give your best to your body, it will return in the same manner. As you could see, our bodies are even more complex than any of us, humans, could ever imagine. There are the tiniest scale processes that can cause the body tremendous problems and diseases if they are stopped in any way. Therefore, it is of utmost importance that we do care about even the smallest processes within our bodies. We will later on focus on the foods that may help you even more to induce autophagy and to maintain your body healthy.

One great 'side effect' of autophagy is that it has several benefits for our immune system. It helps our immune system fight some infective diseases using a couple of different tactics. The first of them is removing microbes directly from the inside of the cells. Also, toxins that are created by different infections are removed. And, finally, immune system response is modulated to infections. Having all of this in mind, we realize how beneficial autophagy is for our entire body system. It not only cleanses our bodies of fats that were accumulated for longer periods of time, but it also does the cleansing on a miniscule level. It cleans our bodies on a cellular and on a molecular level. Those levels are not even visible by our eyes, not without some special equipment. It does its job so well that even our immune system responds better to infections. It can remove toxins, cellular waste, microbes, etc. All of that would remain in our bodies, but, thanks to this amazing process, we are able to get rid of all the harmful components that we accumulated without even knowing.

Another benefit of starting and trying to start off autophagy is longevity. Some studies have shown that autophagy also increases the lifespan. There are studies that were focused on how often autophagy triggers in different life stages. The research has shown that in the early childhood, starting from the birth onwards, the autophagy is the most intense. The body is trying to recover from separating from the mother and the nutrients it's been getting, so the autophagy kicks in and helps the body adapt to a new situation.

As the body gets older, there are less and less of autophagy triggering. However, autophagy doesn't stop once you enter the adulthood. It just starts to kick start less. As one gets older, they are triggering autophagy even less than before. And this is the period many diseases attack the organism, and since it's old and vulnerable, disease may win. Also, there are some indications that people start ageing because their autophagy processes do not work properly or that they are less frequently activated than they should. Some researchers suggest that there is a possibility to be 'forever young' if we figure out the key to make autophagy work when it is supposed to. All of this made researchers think whether it is possible to reduce or even stop ageing. Then, they conducted a series of research and experiments which led them to some conclusions. Of course, the research was not conducted on humans, but animals, like mice. For the experiment they needed to induce autophagy. They tried both drugs that induce autophagy and some other methods, like starvation and exercise.   The research has shown that mice that had autophagy switched on lived longer and they were in better shape. It is believed that their bodies were less intoxicated, and their cells were able to regenerate faster and more frequently. Therefore, they were able to have longer lifespan that the others. On the other hand, there were no researches conducted on humans, so we may not know how this translates to humans. Does it mean that humans too would live longer and have healthier lives? Arguably, yes. Since the autophagy is induced by fasting or intense exercise, there might be even more benefits than we are aware of. Fasting itself reduces fats in the body, as well as exercise does. Intense workouts help your body to stay fit and to build up the muscle mass. All this is very beneficial and healthy for you. Thus, one could say that same would translate to humans as well.

All in all, there are quite a bit of certain evidence that autophagy is indeed a process that will keep your body fit and healthy. With this process turned on, you will benefit in every sense possible. Not only will it regenerate and start off the recycling system within the cells of your body, but it will also remove the fats and all the harmful and negative substances from your body. Wouldn't it be great if one could clean their body from the inside whenever they wanted? Well, you most certainly can! We will discuss all the possibilities in the final, third part of this book. There, you will find out how you can kick start autophagy whenever you want to, and that way clean your body from the inside.

Chapter Six: New Field of Study

♦ ♦ ♦

You most probably could gather this yourself, but here it is: Autophagy is a relatively new field of study. It is known as auto phagocytosis as well. As a word, autophagy was first used in 1963 when Belgian biochemist and cytologist, Christian René de Duve worked on the primeval evidence of how lysosomes were involved in the process of autophagy. There were also some scientists that described the process they've seen under a microscope in 1950s and it matches the description of the process of autophagy perfectly. However, over this long period of time, there were very few researches that dealt with the discovery of this amazing process. The research on this topic was scarce, up until 1990s when Yoshinori Ohsumi started collecting and examining the evidence on its importance. He won the Nobel Prize in 2016 for his contribution to discoveries related to the mechanisms and processes of autophagy. After his interesting discoveries, there were many other scientists that dealt with this field of science and some amazing facts were discovered, some of which we also covered within this book.

In the overall field of autophagy, there are three larger types, and these are: micro autophagy, macro autophagy, and autophagy that is chaperone-mediated. The difference between micro autophagy and macro autophagy is that in micro autophagy, we have cellular components that are directly surrounded by invaginations of a lysosomal membrane. On the other hand, macro autophagy is a process that is seen primarily on cellular level and in this process, damaged or worn out materials within the cells are surrounded by autophagosomes and then recycled for energy or new cell material. The third type of autophagy, which is chaperone-mediated is somewhat different from both of the former types. It is a process that is selective and in this process there is a protein which is called hsc70 chaperone. This protein can recognize and bind to substrates of protein which contain certain motifs of amino acid. This substrate is then carried over to lysosome from where it is translocated across the cellular membrane and this is done by a process that is receptor-mediated.

However, if you research more about autophagy, you will realize that there are much more details and many more types of autophagy that it seems at first. Almost any of the processes that occur in humans' or even other species' bodies are covered with autophagy and there is some type of autophagy involved in that process. Therefore, I will present some of these types, just to give you an insight of how big and encompassing this field of study is. One such type is aggrephagy. Aggrephagy is related to a process where proteins, which are grouped into bigger protein aggregates, are degraded. On a cellular level, these bigger protein aggregates are not as toxic as a larger number of smaller protein aggregates. Next type of autophagy is allophagy. It refers to degradation of mitochondria that is paternally-derived right upon the fertilization that occurs in zygotes. This type can be considered to be a form of another type of autophagy, which is mitophagy. What happens is that sperm mitochondria, which are placed in the central region, are primarily labeled with ubiquitin which is K-63 linked right before the fertilization. This marking is increased right after the fertilization, most probably in order to guarantee successful and fast degradation right before the female and male pronuclei fuse.

There is a type of autophagy that is called exophagy. It is related to nondegradative processes that are involved in secretion of proteins. Heterophagy is another type of autophagy. It represents a process in which extracellular material, which was internalized inside the cell, is degraded, which contrasts with degradation of the intracellular material that is pre-existing. Another big and very important type of autophagy is known as immunophagy. It is the type of autophagy that is involved in the process of creating and maintaining both adaptive and innate immunophagy. There are three subtypes of immunophagy. The first one is involved in processing endogenous or foreign molecules that are immunologically active. The second type is responsible for regulating cell viability as well as cell functions that are closely connected to immunity. And the third type utilizes some specific autophagy (ATG) proteins. However, it doesn't need the entire autophagy process to occur.

Another type of autophagy is lipophagy and it is a process where lipids are metabolically regulated through degrading lipid droplets, which are also known as LDs, via a process known as autophagy. In the end, triglycerides are broken down by fusing with lysosomes into FFA, or free fatty acids. Some studies showed that lipophagy can be used for the regulation of appetite in the hypothalamic cells. It also showed that is the lipolysis is reduced in macrophages, it can cause them to converse into foam cells prematurely, which can promote atherosclerosis. When it comes to bacteria, viruses and parasites, they can be removed by a process that is called xenophagy and it is part of immune defense that is innate.

So, as you could see, there is so much to discover within all of these types. There are so many more types of autophagy, but I don't have the space to elaborate each and every bit into details. You most probably got the gist. There are so many ways in which autophagy helps our bodies that I believe many of them are yet to be discovered. It is not only my opinion. We can see that these experiments are mainly done on small mammals, like mice. Imagine what could possibly be discovered if only someone did extensive researches on how it affects humans. There are some researches, but in the main, one cannot but think how much there is yet to be found and discovered.

All in all, autophagy is not a field of science that was just discovered. It was talked about throughout many decades. However, no one seemed to be interested to dig deeper to discover the real treasures that hide within these processes. Only in the last two decades did scientists revealed some of the secrets that are hidden in the tiniest pieces of humans, cells. Although it is a relatively new field of study, there is a steady base to begin with and then, one can start building secure knowledge about these processes. If we were to talk about each of the types of autophagy, then there would be lots and lots of talk about different cell types, different functions, etc. However, I just wanted to illustrate how vast and diverse this field of study is. It covers pretty much our entire existence. This leads us to a conclusion that autophagy is indeed one of the most important processes that occur within our bodies.

Besides the fact that it still needs to be discovered how things work, but there are also many diseases that are believed to be connected to autophagy or the lack of it. Therefore, it is necessary to be aware that by researching this field of science, one may help humans cure some of the most difficult diseases and disorders. We've already mentioned some of them, but having in mind that autophagy still isn't researched completely and that it possibly affects almost every other process in our bodies, wouldn't it be logical to say that if we do research this field more thoroughly we might see the benefits in the future health of human race. I'm not indicating that one will be able to win it all, and to reverse the process of ageing, but with some additional researches, one might be able to find a solution to one type of disease. Even if there is only one cure to be discovered, it is still worth it, because there are possibly millions of people that are affected by that same disease.

Chapter Seven: Intermittent Fasting

◆ ◆ ◆

Having made clear what autophagy is and how it affects our bodies, we can now turn to the other side which is more relatable to ordinary people and that is discovering how you can trigger autophagy so that it works in your favor. One of the methods that were mostly researched is starvation. There are many experiments that were conducted that proved that autophagy indeed is triggered by starvation process. Therefore, this will be the first method we will be discussing here. Even though starvation and fasting are not the same, there still might be some aspects that are the same or similar, so we will identify fasting as the closest to starvation.

As you probably already know, fasting has been one of the most common practices in many religions and cultures. It has been one of the most important practices for thousands of years for almost all nations and races. Even though the science yet has a long way of discovering all the benefits of fasting and how it affects autophagy activation, fasting was present in almost all parts of human history. This might be the main reason why those people of the past had been living healthy and long lives. They had to hunt, be physically active and eat only when they find the food. This means that they might have been hungry for longer periods, which, again, is the basis of fasting. The manner of fasting is different from culture to culture, but the essence is the same, some particular foods are 'forbidden' for a certain period of time. If we take a bit modern approach to this topic, we will see the resemblance of this ancient type of fasting with the modern type, which is dieting. Doesn't it seem so familiar the way many people take different diets and by doing so, they avoid certain types of food or they even restrain from taking in food at all. I think it is very similar, if not identical, to fasting. Having all this in mind and the fact that starvation is one of the key stressors that can activate autophagy; one has to try to investigate how they can activate this amazing process whenever they feel the need for it. However, this doesn't necessarily mean that you will have to restrain from eating entirely. There are different types of intermittent fasting and diets that are most likely to activate autophagy and they will be discussed here, in this chapter.

16-hour Fast

The first type that we will be discussing in this chapter is 16/8 hour fasting. It is one of the most famous types of fasting that are practiced nowadays. Some people claim that it is the easiest, and the most convenient and most sustainable way for anyone to improve their health and lose weight at the same time. In its essence, this type of intermittent fasting is all about limiting your intake of food and beverages that are high in calories to a timeframe of only eight hours on a daily basis and for the rest of the day, i.e. for the remaining 16 hours you would withhold from food. You can fast this way as often as you want, whether it is every day or once a week. Of course, you may expect the results to be faster and more visible if you practice this fast more often.

This type of intermittent fasting is an easy way to burn fat and lose weight, so it has become very popular in the last couple of years. The reason behind its popularity lies in the fact that it requires a minimal effort from your side, and it is quite easy to adjust to. Almost any lifestyle can be adjusted to it. It is very flexible and less restrictive that other diets. Some of the health benefits of this type of intermittent fasting are enhancing longevity, boosting brain functions and improvement of control over blood sugar. Just from seeing the benefits one can get to a conclusion that it has to be autophagy that is causing all of these great things for our organisms.

To start your 16-hour fast, you will first need to pick a time period in which you will be eating. It would be best to pick any eight hour period of time during the day, since you will be sleeping during night anyways, so all you need to choose is whether you want to have a breakfast or not. If you do, then you can fast from 9-5 and have a breakfast, a lunch some later and an early dinner before you ran out of time. Other options are from 12-8, so that you skip breakfast, but you can have a lunch and a dinner. It all depends on your personal preference. Then, you will pick foods and beverages that you will be consuming during this period and keep away from all foods during the 16-hours fast.

What is important when it comes to the food you will be eating is that you have more of small, but balanced meals filled with nutritious food over this period of time and some snacks in between too. You will need to space these evenly so that the levels of blood sugar are stabilized, and the hunger is kept under control. If you eat foods that are nutrient rich, you will maximize the benefits of this type of fasting. When it comes to which food you can eat, there is plenty to choose from. You can have different kinds of fruits and vegetables, like bananas, apples, different kinds of berries, pears, peaches, oranges, all the leafy greens, broccoli, cucumbers, tomatoes, cauliflower, etc. You can get your proteins from poultry, meat, fish, eggs, seeds, nuts, etc. You can also use so many whole grains like rice, quinoa, barley, oats, etc. and you can take the fats from olive oil, coconut oil and avocado. When it comes to beverages, it is best if you drink water or tea and/or coffee that are unsweetened, because these are calorie free and they can help you get hydrated as well as get control over your appetite. It is important not to eat too much because one can have more negative effects from such behavior than positive ones, so you should beware of that.

Health benefits that are connected to this type of intermittent fasting are numerous. These benefits range from those that are closely connected to autophagy, like cell renewal and regeneration, to some that, again, might be seen as consequences of autophagy, like increased longevity, better control over blood sugar, losing weight, improved brain function, etc. The negative effects can be connected to the current state of your body even before you started fasting. You may feel fatigue or hunger, but this is almost inevitable when dieting. If you do not exaggerate with foods and calories then you will be fine. However, if you do not pay attention to that and eat as much as you can during the eight-hour period, you will most probably gain weight, rather that lose it, and clearly autophagy will not be activated. However, if you do feel a bit weak, you should consult your physician, just to make sure that you can continue with your plan of fasting.

Now, you can see why this method is really popular. It allows you to eat, but within a certain period of time. Its results are visible, regardless whether you want to become healthier or lose weight. And the best results, which are not even visible without some special equipment, are in fact the activation of autophagy which happens on cellular level and regenerates our bodies from the inside. People who have tried this method say that they stick to it for years because it is effective, it gives them results and it is easily adjustable to almost any lifestyle. There are some drawbacks, but those are individual, just like with any other diet regime or fast.

24-hour Fast

Another type of intermittent fasting is 24-hour fasting. Actually, there are some people that call this type a prolonged fasting, whereas others consider it to be intermittent and only fasts that are longer that 48 hours are prolonged. Either way, it is a type of fasting, intermittent or prolonged, and it does come with all of the benefits you would normally get by fasting for certain periods of time.

What may sound difficult is the fact that you are about to fast for 24 hours. This is especially difficult if you haven't done any other type of fasting before. It may seem intimidating to even try, but once you get to find out all the benefits you and your body may be getting from this type of fasting, I'm sure you will at least think about it. Now, previously, I have described what happens to the body in each stage of fasting. There are certain periods of time when you will most definitely feel hunger, but in this type of fasting you can drink water or herbal tea, so do that and your hunger will be easier to live with. From my own experience, fasting for periods longer than 16 hours, like this one, it may be really difficult, especially, if you start thinking about food or how hungry you are. Things will only get worse if you do that. Therefore, you should plan your 24 hours of fasting in detail. This way, you will be busy taking charge of the list or the plan you made and that everything is done on time. You won't have time to think about the hunger. With this type of fasting, people usually plan around one of the meals, for example, they start fasting after breakfast and stop around the same time the next day, or they do it from lunch to lunch or dinner to dinner. You need to choose what fits you the best and try that way. Another important thing is that you start in small steps. If you usually cannot be hungry for longer periods of time, do it gradually. Start by fasting overnight for 12 hours. Let's say you have dinner at 7:30 pm. You only need to keep away from food until 7:30 in the morning the next day. That is easy, you will be sleeping anyways! Then, you just prolong the fasting periods for couple of hours more and more until you feel confident enough to fast for 24 hours. However, even though one may fast for longer periods of time than with this method, it isn't recommended in this method that you repeat this fasting routine more than one or twice a week. You should also pay attention that you take in nutrient rich meals and that there are lots of diverse vitamins, minerals, protein, fibers, and all the good stuff, basically. The meal before starting your fast should be very well balanced and satisfying. Here is a possible schedule for this type of fasting: Let's say you will fast from breakfast to the breakfast the next day. You will have a good, hearty, healthy breakfast and it should keep your stomach from rumbling for almost the entire day. Then, you will run errands for the rest of the day, so that you don't think about the hunger you are feeling. Later in the day, you will get home; spend some time with your family and friends and go to sleep. When you wake up the next day, your fast is finished. Easy peasy, I'd say! This schedule wouldn't be a great match if you hate to go to bed with an empty stomach or you are not really a morning person or the breakfast one either. That is why you should analyze and plan according to your preferences. Of course, during this period of time, you can drink water or some unsweetened herbal tea. Some researchers say that coffee should be avoided because of the caffeine that may cause a mess inside the body, while others say that some other ingredients of the coffee can actually induce autophagy and give you a boost of autophagy activation. I would suggest you try and see for yourself what suits you and your body the best. It is a fact that the body is much more sensitive to caffeine than it is when you're not fasting. However, it is best that everyone tests it out for themselves.

Now, when it comes to the benefits that this type of fasting has for your health, they are numerous. You probably guessed it; it induces autophagy. That is what makes the whole difference in your overall health. Autophagy will fight against cell defects that might cause cancer and some mental disorders, it might increase your lifespan, and it protects your heart and so many other good stuff. It is not yet proven when autophagy gets activated in humans, but some studies suggest that it might be between 16 and 24 hours of fasting. However, since it is not proven in any way yet, one cannot be sure. Therefore, we should strive to fast a bit longer just to make sure that we get to that stage when autophagy is activated, and our cells do recycle the harmful materials and that they do regenerate. Another important thing for this type of fasting is that, just like with any other, you should make sure that you eat healthy, fat free, carbohydrates free meals. That way, you will give a different chance to your cells that have worked hard to recycle and regenerate. And, after all, you don't want all that effort to be done for nothing.

The 5:2 Diet: Fast for 2 Days per Week

The name says it for itself. The 5:2 diet is a plan of dieting in which you eat regularly for five days and you fast for two days a week. So, this diet is very simple. Basically, you don't need to count calories for five days in a week. You can eat whatever you want. On the two days that you're fasting, you are allowed eat, but up to a limit of 500-600 calories, the first one being the limit for women and the latter for men. Another rule to this type of fasting/dieting is that these two days should not be consecutive, i.e. there should be at least one day that separates them.

You may ask yourself, if you do not change your regular eating regime during a five day period and you do not change it in the fasting period, and only reduce it to 500-600 calories, are you going to have any benefits? Well, it depends on what you eat on a normal, regular basis. If you are eating healthy, balanced meals every day, you won't have problems. However, if you are eating junk food all the time and in this way make up for all the food you have missed in the fasting days, then, you will most probably gain weight instead of losing it. I suppose that it is not anyone's goal to do so. So, if you are having an unhealthy meal plans, you will probably miss out on all the benefits this and any other type of fasting yields.

When it comes to the benefits of this type of fasting, there isn't much research that was done on this topic. However, whatever is applicable to other types of fasting, one may definitely say for this one too. If you remember, when we talked about fasting and the process of autophagy, it is said that the maximal amount of food that you can eat is 500 calories within 24 hours. This is exactly what you would do with this type of fasting. You will eat just enough so that you don't feel hungry or weak. So, basically, even with this approach, you should be able to induce autophagy and help your body restore energy from within and to activate the recycling process within your cellular and molecular levels. Of course, this may depend on other factors as well. For example, you will not lose weight, nor it is possible to activate autophagy if you are eating lots of carbohydrates and sugar. On the other hand, you will most probably have all the benefits that fasting can bring you if you have normal, balanced and diverse meals.

There are some studies that have shown that this type of diet can definitely cause weight loss and that it is very good in the reduction of insulin levels as well as in the overall improvement in insulin sensitivity. Another diet which is similar to this one, the 4:3 diet, or fasting every other day, has shown great results in the reduction of insulin resistance, seasonal allergies, asthma, hot flashes caused by menopause, heart arrhythmias and many more. Other studies have shown that it helps people reduce fat, lose weight, but there is no loss of the muscle mass. It is a relatively easy to adapt to diet plan, so it is readily available to everyone. If you feel encouraged enough, then, you can start following 4:3 diet plan, which is quite similar. Of course, it is very important that you do not make up for the missed calories during the fasting days because there will be no results if you do that. You will not lose any weight if you make up for the lost calories, in fact, you may even gain some.

When it comes to food, there is not a rule as to what you can and cannot eat of your fasting days. You should probably opt for healthy, nutritious, protein and fiber rich meals that will keep you full for longer periods of time. Still, you should keep it under 500/600 calories, just to make sure you are on the right track. Now, you can choose to divide these 500/600 calories however you want during the day, but there are two ways that are more common. You can either choose to have three small meals that would include breakfast, lunch and dinner or you can skip breakfast and just have two meals, i.e. lunch and dinner which would then be a little bit bigger. It, again, all depends on your preference and you can choose to have just one big meal, though, that wouldn't be very smart to do, since you can divide these meals during the day. You can have vegetables, fish, eggs, lean meat, yogurt with fruits, different kinds of soups, etc. When it comes to beverages, it is best to drink plain water or sparkling water. You can have some tea or coffee, just like with any other diet.

Now we come to the question if this type of fasting/dieting can induce autophagy. In my opinion, yes, it can. If you do follow the rules and do no overeat during the days when you're not fasting, you can achieve your goal of activating autophagy and help your body regenerate and possibly rejuvenate. Once again, just like the 16-hour fast, this one isn't too difficult to incorporate in any lifestyle. You can experiment and see what suits you and your needs best and go with it. Just have in mind all the basics that need to be taken into account and you'll get there, don't worry.

The Warrior Method

Yeah, the name itself is a bit scary, I must admit. This diet or fasting method was introduced by a man who was a military member Ori Hofmekler in 2001, hence the name, warrior method. He was a member of Special Forces of Israel, but then he made a transition to explore health, nutrition and fitness. He designed this fasting pattern to resemble the regime of warriors from past times, where they would eat very small amounts of food during the day, but when the night comes, they would have big feasts. The founder himself says that this type of fasting is not based on any scientific researches, but only on his observations and beliefs. It is said to boost health, looks and performances. This method actually encourages you to eat very small amounts of food during 20-hour time period and then feast on whatever your heart desires for four remaining hours. Many people think that this diet is to rigorous and unnecessary, but people who have actually fasted in this manner say that it is really beneficial, and they have been repeating the routine for many times later on. People that have tried this method of fasting say that it is good for burning fat, improving concentration, boosting energy levels and stimulating cellular repair.

Since there is very little difference between some other forms of fasting and this one, one may not say that the benefits of other fasting methods will not be applicable to this type of fasting. It is very similar to 16:8 fasting method, the only difference being the fact that you would fast four hours longer than in the 16:8 method. However, there are diets that require even longer periods of fasting, like 24-hour fast and some other, so this method isn't the longest. Therefore, it would be unfair to say that if this method is not researched that it does not have any benefits for your health. It does have many benefits, just like any other fasting method. One could claim that this method would be better candidate for autophagy activation since the body is under stress of starvation for longer period of time and therefore it has to make up for the loss of energy and nutrients. The only problematic part of this way of fasting may be the fact that people are encouraged to eat everything they want. Therefore, they could potentially ruin their fast by consuming foods that are not healthy in one way or the other. Some studies have shown that in a similar environment like this one here, people have experienced the loss of weight even though they have been eating over the period of four hours, whereas other people ate the same amount of food during the entire day. These people, who had only one meal a day, experienced a reduction in fat mass and an increase of muscle mass. Now that we have this study in mind, one cannot help but ask themselves how is that even possible? To eat all you want at night and the amount can equal to what they would regularly eat throughout one day and yet lose weight? Interesting, right? Many diets recommend not to eat in the late afternoon at all because those meals are the ones which make you gain weight. What is different in this case? Well, you guessed it! Autophagy is what happens here. Since you would fast for 20 hours during the day, with only small amounts of calories taken in, your body would be forced to work hard and activate the process of autophagy in your body, which would in turn result in weight loss. Your body is then, in the process of fasting, forced to use fats as a fuel for energy and for all other processes that occur inside your body, so you will most probably lose weight as a result of fasting. When it comes to foods that you would break your fast with, again, it is not recommended to devour candies, sugar and carbohydrates. Of course, you can make up for the loss, but you will get to your objective much faster if you completely rule out these from your diet.

When it comes to other health benefits from this type of fasting, they are numerous. As with many other types of intermittent fasting, you will be improving your brain's health by practicing intermittent fasting. When you are fasting, some inflammatory markers are reduced, which would otherwise impact your learning and memory in a negative way. This, as well as some studies that have shown that fasting reduces the possibility of Alzheimer's disease, are done mostly on animals, so in order to confirm it, there should be many studies done on humans to confirm the theory true. However, since many other improvements have proven to be true, we might say that when this theory is examined, it will most probably be true also. Other health benefits are lowering the level of inflammations and better control of blood sugar. When fasting intermittently, one might experience lowering of blood sugars, which is also known as hypoglycemia. Even though lower blood sugar is generally good, it may lead to some complications, so it is best to consult with your doctor before you start fasting, especially this type of fasting.

The negative side of this type of fasting is that it may be very difficult to follow, especially if you want to enjoy your daily activities with friends and family. Then, there are some groups of people that should avoid this type of fasting, like pregnant and nursing women, children, people with diabetes type one, heart failures or some cancers, underweight persons or those with some eating disorders, or some athletes. Another issue that might appear is with women. They may experience change in hormones, which in turn may affect some other aspects of their life, like sleeping, mood, menstrual changes and disturbances in reproductive health. Luckily, these changes are not what every woman experiences, but it is good to have in mind if it happens, so that you know how to react.

When it comes to fasting itself, there is a three-week schedule that you should follow. The first one is a detox stage where you should be removing all the toxins from your body, the second one is called high fat and it is similar to the first one, only difference being that it includes meat and nuts also and the third one is where you conclude fat loss and here, you will alternate between days with high level of carbohydrates and days with high level of proteins.

When you finish these two weeks, you can start over again or you can skip the first week and continue from the second. Also, each day is divided into two phases, one of undereating for 20 hours and the other where you are overeating for four hours. This method may be good to use, and you can possibly try and thrive on it, but there are so many strict rules to follow and the time period of fasting is pretty long. Also, there are no restrictions with regards of the number of calories you may consume during the four hour period of overeating, nor is there a number of calories you can take in during the undereating phase. It seems like a vague guide as to how you can fast, but without precise boundaries. This may be problematic for some people, especially those that might feel that they need to eat more because the undereating period is too long. All in all, this method of fasting may be great for some people and it may give great results, but for most of the people, it may be too restricting and maybe a bit too long. But, then again, without putting your body under stress, you won't get the benefits of autophagy and this should be your goal. In the end, whatever you choose, please contact your doctor so that you are sure that you can fast for a period of time you choose.

Meal Skipping

One of the easiest and most beginner friendly methods of fasting is definitely this one, meal skipping. Basically, you will eat normally as you would, but if you feel like you are not hungry and that you could easily go without that meal, you can just skip that meal and eat when the next meal period comes. So, there is no schedule to follow or anything. You will feel your body's needs and act accordingly. If you feel hungry, then, you will fulfill that need. If you don't feel hungry, you will skip that meal and that's it. However, if you add seriousness to this method of intermittent fasting, then, you may develop your own schedule. For example, there are some people that don't enjoy having breakfast or they think it is too early to eat as soon as they get up. They might skip breakfast and have the rest of the meals as they normally would. Likewise, many people do not want to eat dinner too late, so they would rather have their lunch a bit later in the afternoon and skip dinner altogether. And that is fine also. With this method of fasting, you may pick whatever schedule you are comfortable with. On the other hand, you don't have to follow a schedule at all. If you feel that you are not hungry, you can just skip the meal and that's it. However, other meals should be well balanced, with plenty of nutrients, proteins and fibers.

Regardless of what you may choose when it comes to skipping meals, there are so many different expert opinions as to how it may be even harmful to fast or diet this way. There are so many reasons why you should not skip meals whenever you don't feel like eating and one of them is the feeling of tiredness and dizziness. This may occur due to low blood sugar levels and it is most often because there is no schedule to rely on. Your body needs a routine around which you will function. Even if you are fasting for longer periods of time, you still have a schedule and your body adapts to it. However, if you skip breakfast today, dinner tomorrow, lunch on some other day, it gives your body a completely new message.

Apart from that, one may feel like they have missed something by skipping a meal and then have the urge to compensate for the loss. There also might be a change in hormones so that you won't feel when you are hungry and when you are full, which might lead to overeating and obesity. It may also affect your mood since your body will run out of glucose which helps you boost your mood. Of course, it happens to everyone that they skip a meal sometimes and it is okay if it happens from time to time. But, if you are doing it on purpose and all the time, it may become a problem rather than a solution to your problem. Plus, if you look at this type of fasting/dieting from the aspect of autophagy induction, you may notice that there is less possibility to trigger the activation of autophagy using this method. This is so because you won't be fasting for such long periods of time that it will cause immediate stress to your body. However, if breakfast or dinner are the meals you will skip, there might be somewhat longer periods of time without eating, so there is a chance for autophagy activation to occur. On the other hand, there is no planning, scheduling or anything, so, you are not sure when is the next meal you are going to skip. It may be good for you, if you are not overeating at the next meal and if you are eating healthy, balanced meals. On the other side, if you don't have any plans, if you are eating a lot and unhealthy, then this method may be very harmful for you. The bottom line is that you should plan and take into consideration everything when you want to fast for your health.

Alternate Day Fasting

From the easiest fasting methods to maybe the most difficult, here is another extreme. If you are looking for an extreme fasting method, alternate day fasting (ADF) is one of them. It is a method where you fast for 36 hours and then eat for 12 hours. Fasting for 36 hours is done in several ways. Some people fast with no intakes. Others just drink water and coffee, while some others consume food up until 500 calories per fasting day. This depends on the person and how much hunger and thirst they can handle. If you look at it as a full fasting method, it is the most extreme method of fasting presented here. It lasts for a longer period of time and it can become very difficult to follow. During the 12 hours you can eat as much as you want. And then, you have the full cycle and start a new one.

There was a study conducted on 60 people who were all healthy and had normal weight. They were divided into two groups, those that were fasting and those that were not. They measured the parameters throughout the four week period. The results have shown many benefits that are connected to one's health and longevity. Some of the findings indicate that those people who practice fasting might be living longer. These results aren't shockingly good because many people expected similar results from what has been discovered from experiments on animals. This just proved those earlier findings to be true of humans too. These health benefits may be closely connected to a process that is of utmost importance in our bodies and that is autophagy. As you could see from the previous chapters, autophagy is seen to be connected to longevity and regeneration, as well as weight loss. In order for autophagy to activate, one does not have to fast on no calories; you may take in some calories, but still, not more than 500 calories per day. Weight loss, cellular regeneration and recycling are guaranteed. As with 24 hour fasting, you get all the benefits of fasting, which also include autophagy activation.

Experts and researchers warn that this type of diet, just like the warrior method, is not for everyone. It consists of long periods of fasting on no calories to as some experts suggest 500 calories. Experts say that it is not necessary to fast on no calories for such a long period of time, but that one can consume up to 500 calories per day and still have the same effects as if they were fasting without any calorie intake. They also suggest that this type of fasting is a bit stricter than the others and that therefore it may not be suitable for everyone. The period of fasting is extremely long and therefore it might affect some people's health and overall state in a negative way. However, if one is fighting with weight loss and they realize that this method is helping them lose weight as they imagined it would, then this is the right method for them. Anyway, this method is definitely suitable for longer periods of time and one cannot adjust their lifestyle according to this type of fasting, like it might be possible with some other types. Additionally, one may experience some other difficulties with their health, so overall, if you are not feeling well, you should quit this type of fasting. All in all, alternate day fasting method is an effective one. It will definitely help you out in the activation of autophagy and regenerate and recycle from within, but it is also not for everyone due to long periods of fasting and the complications that may arise from that issue.

Having reviewed all of these different types of fasting, one may come to several conclusions. These are: if you are fasting for periods longer than 12 hours, you are most likely going to induce autophagy, which is a process that happens within our bodies on a cellular and molecular levels and it helps our bodies stay healthy. Autophagy is the most important process because it will clean out and recycle all the waste that has been collected within our system. Also, it is an important factor in prevention of many diseases. With all of these types of fasting, you will most probably lose weight, reduce calorie intake, and maybe get more disciplined, etc. Health benefits are numerous, such as better brain power, reduced inflammation, prevention of many diseases, etc. This all works on the basis that you initiate the process of autophagy and the organism itself will do its job. And one way to initiate the process is by starvation or, in other words, fasting. One could never imagine the complexity of processes that occur on such small levels, but science has proven it and there are more and more studies that confirm and even discover some new insights into the world of autophagy.

Chapter Eight: Regular Exercise

◆ ◆ ◆

We have discussed one way of activating and regulating autophagy and that is starvation or in our case, a modification of starvation which is called fasting. This is a great and easy way to activate this awesome process and improve your overall health. However, there is another way of inducing autophagy and that is with exercise. This is because exercise puts your body into stress. When you exercise, you actually cause microscopic damages to your muscles. Then, your body activates autophagy in order to fix problems up and heal those micro tears that were caused by exercise. Your cells begin the process of autophagy to clean up all the negative components and to build up new, stronger bonds and tissues. This process in fact makes your muscles more damage resistant and stronger. If you do exercise regularly, you will actually help your body cleanse itself from the inside.

There are now several studies both on animals and on humans that proved how exercise increases the number of autophagosomes inside cells. Exercise does not just help you build up your muscles, but it also helps you clean up your body. A study has shown that mice which were running on treadmills for about 30 minutes had a significant increase of autophagosomes, which are actually responsible for carrying out the process of autophagy. Then, they observed them until they were running for about 80 minutes and it just showed them that the number of autophagosomes continued increasing. This got the researchers intrigued and some of them began asking themselves what happens to humans when they exercise.

Of course, exercising is very beneficial, regardless of whether we look at it from the perspective of autophagy or not. It helps you lose excess weight, tone and build up the muscle mass, remove toxins from your body and all other great things. However, if we do look at it from the perspective of a process such as autophagy, is it fair if we say that autophagy just helps us cleanse our bodies? It actually does much more to our bodies and most probably, it is mainly responsible for all the benefits I named earlier. As we have seen from the previous scientific works, autophagy can help us lose weight by burning the fats instead of carbohydrates and sugars. It can help you build your muscle mass by renewing the bonds and regenerating the cells that were damaged by exercising. And most certainly, it does remove toxins by identifying the negative compounds within cells and recycling them into new cell material or energy.

A recent study was actually done on humans and it has shown some impressive results. The study was conducted on fourteen males who were all healthy and physically active. The research was done using exercise like cycling and sprint. Measurements were taken before, during and two hours after the exercise. Also, biopsies of muscle were taken at all three stages and also at the stage of resting after training. The results showed that there are many differences before and in the stages during and after the exercise. They have shown that exercising has increased autophagy markers in skeletal muscles of humans in a period of two hours right after the exercise took place and the body was in a state of recovery. The research also suggested that exercise that lasted for eight weeks has increased the autophagy capacity as well as regulation of mitophagy. Therefore, these recent findings have provided evidence that workouts and such trainings can and will regulate the process of autophagy in the skeletal muscles of humans. This study concludes that the results they got from the research suggest that even one exercise session increased the number of autophagosomes, and that one can increase the autophagy capacity and the regulation of mitophagy in the skeletal muscles of humans with exercise trainings.

Of course, this isn't the only study that was done on humans and with regards to exercise. There was another study which had the participants divided into two groups, one that was fasting and one that was eating regularly. Both of the groups were subjected to some intense exercises. The results have shown that regardless of whether the participants were eating or not, the intensity of the exercises was the one which increased the number of autophagosomes significantly or not. The measurements have shown that the increase is the same both in those that were fasting and those that were eating, which leads to a conclusion that exercise might be even more important than eating or fasting.

Types of Exercises

When it comes to exercises that may help you activate the process of autophagy, they are really numerous. The studies were observing running on a treadmill in mice and cycling and sprint in humans. So, there are such exercises that you can do in a gym and use all the equipment that is there, and you may help your body to induce autophagy and benefit from it. The studies that have included cycling and sprint actually talk about 60 minutes of exercising. It generally isn't much, but if you are intensely cycling or running, you may feel fatigue.

However, there are some other types of exercise that you can do which don't require much of equipment. These are endurance exercises. The first and probably one of the most famous is the plank. In this exercise you will lay down on the ground on your stomach. You will lean on your elbows and lift up your hips so that you rely only on your elbows and tips of your toes. Elbows should be standing at a 90 degree angle and your back and legs should be tightened. You should stay this way for 30 to 40 seconds and then relax. Of course, some people won't be able to endure that long, but you can increase each day by five seconds until you get to that stage. Repeat for as many times you want, optimally you should do at least five repetitions of the plank.

The next type of exercise is squats. This is also a familiar exercise type. Basically, you need to set your feet a bit wider than the width of your shoulders. Then, you will lower your body in a squat position, where your knees should be placed at a 90 degrees angle. Then, you will push yourself up and repeat in sets of 25 or as many you are able to do. The next endurance exercise is walking lunge. In this exercise you will stand with your feet apart and then step forwards with one leg. Then, lower your body so that your back leg is near the ground. Push yourself upwards and do the same with the other leg. Repeat for as many times you are able to, optimally several sets of 25 to 30 lunges. The next endurance exercise is pushups. It is similar to plank. The beginning is the same. You will place your body in a plank position and then lower your body close to the ground and then push it upwards. Repeat as many times you feel you can do. The last endurance exercise is sit-ups. With sit-ups, you will be laying on your back, with your legs slightly bent. Your hands should be under your head. Then, you will push your upper part of your body towards your knees and back to the lying position. Repeat this for as many times you are able to. Of course, you may begin with five repetitions of each and then, each day, you can increase by one or two more repetitions until you get to the goal number of repetitions during one set and then move to doing more sets. That is if you are not exercising regularly. If you are, then, you can do as many sets of repetitions you feel your body can handle and by causing your body to be under stress you can be sure to help your body to start the process of autophagy that will eventually help you in so many ways.

Other things that you can do daily, that don't actually have the name exercise written all over them, but still may be identified as such are walking up the stairs instead of taking an elevator. You probably know that there are also exercises that are designed to mimic this activity and that include a stepping stool. Why do that when you can climb up or down the stairs for several floors and get the benefits of such exercise without even thinking that you are working out. Next, you can walk instead of driving anywhere. Nowadays, everyone is so used to driving their car even to the nearest point in place they need to go. Stop doing that! You can walk instead. This will become extremely helpful especially if your job requires you to sit all your working hours and then, even when you get out of work, you still sit, but in your car. Change this habit into a new one, where you will walk to work, to the shop, to a cinema, wherever you want to go, because those steps will eventually add up and you will be moving and building your muscles just by moving from one place to another. Also, you can force yourself to stand more because it can burn more calories as opposed to sitting, it can also improve one's posture and it usually makes you work more actively than when you are sitting comfortably.

You can also include running sessions or some other exercises that will put some pressure on your muscles. Ideally, you would want to choose exercises that will put your body under a stress so that it will activate the process of autophagy as a reaction to that stressful environment. If you are a person that exercises regularly, then you are probably familiar with so many exercises that you can actually incorporate in your training sessions and you will most definitely benefit from them. However, if you are not exercising regularly, you should consider taking some time to get yourself involved in exercising sessions and training because there are so many proofs that exercise is indeed good for our bodies and you should leave out a period of time during the day to work out and help your body regenerate. As you could see, some studies suggest that exercise is even more important than the diet when it comes to autophagy induction and improvement. This does not have to be true for each and every person, but there are big chances that if you do exercise regularly and start intermittent fasting for some periods during a week or a month, you will benefit more than if you just do one of these things. After all, everyone is completely aware of all the benefits exercise can have to our overall health and condition. However, if you have any health issues, you should better first consult your doctor about starting a program of exercising and if they approve, only if they do approve, you should start exercising. Otherwise, you should obey if they say that it might be risky or that you should not work out at all for some reason. Your current health is all that matters. Of course, if there is a way to improve your health, then, you should go for it, but if there is any chance that you will ruin your health even more, then it is best to avoid such things.

All in all, there are some very convincing evidences that exercising may give a boost to your autophagy process and regulate the mitophagy process. This is especially important because the studies were done on humans, as well as some animals and the results were almost identical. Humans that were subjected to exercises have shown that there are many more indicators of autophagy during and after the session than there were before the exercises. This proves that exercises can be one of the inducers of autophagy, which is important in case of some disease treatments, weight loss, etc.

Chapter Nine: Adjusting Your Diet

◆ ◆ ◆

In order to activate and regulate the process of autophagy, it is necessary to be in constant connection to what is going on in your body. You may notice that you will need to be more physically active, as suggested in the previous chapter or that you are going to need to adjust your daily diet as well. Studies have shown that both what you eat and what you do during the day may affect the activation and regulation of autophagy. However, it is not necessary to induce the process of autophagy every day. You may do it, but it is also fine if you do it occasionally. We already talked about all the different kinds of exercise you can do in order to induce autophagy process. You were made familiar with how exercise induced autophagy works and what it does to your body. Hopefully, that motivated you to start working out regularly. When it comes to your diet, you may add some simple changes, such as reducing the number of calories you take each day or removing some types of food out of your diet completely, which will be further discussed. All in all, these are the two major changes that you can do to make your body and life much better. Now, when it comes to different diets, there are two that might be distinguished from all others. These are low carb diet and intermittent fasting diet. We will now discuss each of these and what types of food you can consume in both of these cases.

Low Carb Diet

Low carb diet is basically a diet with very low to none intake of carbohydrates. Carbohydrates are usually found in bread, pasta and sugary foods. This type of dieting is also called LCHF diet, which means that it is low in carbs and high in fats. Others also call it keto diet. It is called keto diet because when you reduce the number of carbohydrates and sugars, your body is forced to burn fat and as a result it produces ketone bodies or ketones in your liver, which are then used for energy and other processes.

In this type of diet, you are encouraged to stay away from sugars and starches, while you can eat all the fats you want. Contrary to the popular belief that fats are dangerous and damaging to our bodies, it has been proven that it is the carbohydrates that may cause our health to worsen. The increased intake of carbohydrates might be the reason why obesity is so epidemic-like. There were many campaigns of low fat foods which are in fact filled with carbohydrates and sugars, and as a result there has been an increase of overly obese people. It may be a coincidence, but it may actually have some really strong connections to that. On the other hand, when we talk about fats, there are different kinds of fats and those that are natural can be considered to be good for you.

When you omit starches and sugary foods from your diet, your body will start burning the fats, you will feel less hungry and therefore you will reduce the food intake and as a result you will be losing weight. Also, it is much easier to control your blood sugar level with this type of diet. There are also many other health benefits that were proven to be connected to this type of dieting.

When it comes to what kinds of food you are allowed to eat, these are meats, eggs, fish, vegetables that are low in carbohydrates, mostly those that grow above the ground and fats like butter. As we have already mentioned, you should avoid foods that are rich in sugars and starches. In this type of dieting, there is no need to count the number of calories you are going to take, just eat whenever you are hungry and stop whenever you feel full. This type of diet is not safe for everyone, though. People that have diabetes or high blood pressure should first consult their doctor about starting this type of diet. Pregnant and breastfeeding women should also be careful if they are planning to start this or any other type of diets. Of course, if you do not have any health issues and you want to try this type of diet, but you feel a little bit insecure if it is going to affect your health, you can always talk to your doctor about it and see what advice you are going to get. If you have problems with obesity, this diet is definitely going to help you with that problem.

However, regardless of how much effort you take into planning and cooking, you may end up having some carbohydrates anyways. It is almost impossible to have a diet that is free from carbohydrates. But, in order to stay within the keto or ketogenic diet, you need to lower the amount of carbohydrates to an amount that is less than twenty grams during one day. This is a strict ketogenic diet and it has most results, and having autophagy in mind, this is when it will be the most effective. Then, there is moderate low carb diet that is limited from twenty to fifty grams of carbohydrates per one day. And then, there is the liberal type which is limited to 50 to 100 grams of carbs per day. As I already said, the results are the best if one is following a strict keto diet and it will most definitely reflect in weight loss and the control of blood sugar. Therefore, you may want to start off with the strict type which will limit your carb intake very much. You may continue this way until you realize that you have reached your goal in weight loss and then switch to some more liberal type where you can have some carbs here and there. This way, you will still feed healthy, but you will be able to indulge in some other kinds of food from time to time.

You will be allowed to eat meat, including beef, lamb, poultry, and pork. You don't have to avoid fats from the meat. It is best if they are organic. Same thing is with eggs, you can eat all kinds of eggs. You can also eat all kinds of fish and also seafood. When it comes to fats, you can use butter, olive oil, coconut oil and practically all natural fats. You can eat all the vegetables that grow above the ground. When it comes to dairy products, you can consume all of them, even better if you choose those with higher fat percentage. You can also eat nuts and some berries as long as you keep the amounts limited. As for drinks, it is best to drink water or sparkling water. You can also drink unsweetened tea and coffee. You can add whipped cream or milk to your coffee or some coconut fat or butter. The bottom line is that you don't have to be careful about the fats at all, just avoid carbs and you'll be fine. When it comes to foods that need to be avoided in this type of diet, you should avoid sugars, including chocolate, pastries, artificial sweeteners, ice cream, cakes, drinks that contain lots of sugar; starches, including potatoes, fries, chips, bread, rice, pasta, cereals, etc. If you are not too careful about the amounts of carbohydrates you consume, you can take some reasonable amounts of root vegetables also. Saturated fats should be avoided, as well as beer. When it comes to fruits, you can eat fruits as natural candies, but you should limit the amounts since they are full of carbohydrates.

Health benefits of this type of diet are numerous, from weight loss to reducing blood sugar. It can also help your guts become more settled and less irritated. You will also be able to reduce sweets and lose fats from your body. Besides from these, many people reported improvements in their skin, blood pressure, headaches, fertility, mental health, etc. when you look at all the benefits, who wouldn't want to try out this amazing diet that brings you nothing but good. As a matter of fact, you may be benefiting from this lifestyle and diet change in the long run because there is some evidence that this and such types of diets can actually affect longevity and thus increase your life span.

Intermittent Fasting Diet

We have already discussed different types and fasting methods, but there are still some key aspects of fasting that need to be covered. Many people would say that fasting is identical to starvation and that in fact is starvation. However, this is not true. Starvation is not voluntary action that one decides to have for a day or two. It is a set of circumstances that a person is left without any food sources. On the other hand, people voluntarily decide to fast for a certain period of time for their own health or any other reason they may have. Starvation represents a lack of available foods and it may result in very bad health conditions and even death. On the other hand, you have fasting, where people do have the food, but they choose not to consume it. If intermittent fasting is done in the right way, it should never cause suffering or death.

If you look at it, there are so many forms of intermittent fasting, that in general, one can say that fasting does not have any specific duration or a rule that needs to be followed. However, we did cover quite a few types of intermittent fasting, and almost all of those types do have a certain periods of time when you are allowed to eat and periods of time when you are fasting. An interesting word in

English is breakfast, meaning that you breakfast with that meal. Since most of the people sleep during the night and not eat all night, it makes sense that you break your fast with that meal. This just goes to show that fasting used to be a part of everyday life back in the past, only that people did not know about all the benefits fasting brings to you. One such benefit is losing weight by burning fat. Much like with the low carb diet, your body turns to fat deposits in your body and burns it to get the energy your body needs. This means that even when you are fasting, you can get into state of ketosis and your liver will eventually produce ketones that will be used for energy.

To break it down into simple, easy to understand explanation, your body can be in either one of the two states, first one being fed state when insulin levels are high and the other one which is when the insulin is low, i.e. the state of fasting. When insulin levels are high, mTOR sends the cells signals to grow and duplicate and generally your body spends that to create energy. When you fast, your insulin levels are low and mTOR signals the cells to start cleaning up and recycling materials that will be used for energy production. This way, your body will burn fat and make you fit without even doing anything.

Apart from losing weight, burning fat and lowering blood sugar levels, there are some other health benefits that come from intermittent fasting. By reducing the level of blood sugar, there is a possibility of reversing type two of diabetes. However, if you do have diabetes, you should first consult your doctor before you start fasting, since your current therapy probably won't work anymore. Another benefit of fasting is an improvement of mental health, concentration and clarity of mind in particular. This does not happen to everyone who is fasting, but there is a possibility that your energy will increase, especially in the last couple of hours of fasting. Of course, with the right type or method of fasting, you are most probably going to trigger the process of autophagy, which will lead to many other health benefits, such as longer lifespan, lowered blood pressure and blood cholesterol. With autophagy, you will actually start the process of cellular cleansing, so that you will clean your body of toxins, bad cellular material and all other harmful components. This, in turn, may result in prevention of many illnesses, such as cancer, and some mental disorders, like Parkinson's and Alzheimer's disease. Also, another benefit that is closely connected to autophagy is reducing the inflammation. This just shows how beneficial is to leave your body to work through the fat deposits once more and not to feed it all the time. The benefits are numerous. Imagine how many more benefits are there yet to be discovered when researches on humans take place a bit more frequently. I am sure that there is plenty of information that is still hiding from the researchers until they do perform studies on humans.

There are several tips and tricks that might help you out when you are fasting. For example, if you have never fasted, you can start with some light fasting methods that can easily fit into any lifestyle. You can start with 16:8 fasting method. There are so many examples how to organize your day to have the full benefits of fasting and still have a social life and everything else. For example, you can start your fast from 7 pm. You can go to bed early, then, in the morning, you will skip breakfast and around 11 am you can start eating again. Once you see that this is not difficult to do, you can increase gradually by one hour until you get to more rigorous methods of fasting. These stricter methods may seem too harsh, but these are the ones you may benefit the most from. However, if you do decide that you cannot fast for periods longer than 16 hours that is fine too. You can also switch to low carb diet and boost this process up even more. Many people ask themselves if they should do exercise while they are fasting. Well, generally, you can. But it always comes down to how you feel. If you feel dizzy or low on energy, maybe you should not exercise while you are fasting. That having said, some studies have shown that people that exercised while they were fasting had a bigger number of autophagosomes than those that did not exercise. Having that in mind, you can try it for the sake of health. However, if you feel weak, it is better not to work out while you are fasting.

When it comes to foods and beverages that are good for you while you are fasting, there are many different opinions. Preferences vary from one method of intermittent fasting to the other. A general rule is that you should eat balanced, healthy meals that are full of nutrients, fibers and proteins. This actually resembles the food pattern that is typical of low carb diet. The fact that low carb diet itself can do so many good things to your body urges you to think what would happen if the benefits of fasting and low carb diet would add up. The best possible results can be obtained using this method. However, there are some intermittent fasting methods like the warrior method where you are encouraged to eat whatever you want during the overeating period of four hours. All in all, the key is to give your body all the nutrients it needs in order to function in the best way possible.

Other tips on how to go through the day are simple and easy to follow, such as to drink plenty of water. Coffee and tea are also allowed. You should keep yourself busy so that even if you feel hungry, you will ignore it and continue with fasting. Even though many people think that hunger will accumulate during the day, it actually does not. It may come in several waves, but if you keep yourself busy they will go just as they came. Do not quit after a day of fasting. You should try to fast for at least a month to see if that give you the desired results. Remember that none of the diets makes your weight go away overnight. Another great advice is to eat low carb food in between the periods of fasting. This will reduce hunger and you will fast a lot easier. The greatest tip of them all is do not binge eat, especially on unhealthy foods after you finish fasting. This will give you the worst possible outcome. There will be no results to be proud of.

Since a person can never be cautious enough, I would once again ask you to please contact your doctor before you enroll in any of the given methods of fasting or dieting or even exercise. Also, even when your doctor gives you approval you've been wanting, please listen to your body and the signals it gives you. If you feel like something is wrong, immediately stop with the procedure and again, talk to your doctor about it. Of course, you will be experiencing episodes of hunger and constipation because the intake of food is reduced. You can use laxatives if you feel discomfort. Another common side effect is headache. It appears on first couple of days, but it will disappear right after your body gets accustomed to the new routine. You can take some more salt to help you out with headaches. You may also experience dizziness, muscle cramps and heartburn. You can help yourself with some sparkling water. All in all, if you feel good, do fast because it will help your body immensely.

Conclusion

◆ ◆ ◆

As you are aware by now, autophagy is really one of the most important processes that occur within our bodies. It is of utmost importance for staying healthy and fit, and most importantly alive. If there weren't for a process like autophagy, our cells would gather too many harmful and negative components that they couldn't work properly, and they would most probably enter into state of decay. Therefore, in order for us to stay healthy and alive, we need to crack the code to how to keep this process in a good state. It is very important that our cells do cleanse themselves from the damaged organelles and misfolded proteins. It is important for number of reasons. Many people start fasting or dieting or even exercising because they are overweight or they want to increase the muscle mass, but, in my opinion, there are some other things that need to be on top of our priority list. The first of them should be our health. You were presented results of some studies, which have shown that autophagy can be used in the process of cancer treatment, as well as in the prevention of this cruel disease. Besides from cancer, there are other diseases and disorders that may develop from the lack of function of autophagy. Among them are neurodegenerative diseases, like Alzheimer's and Parkinson's disease, as well as some metabolic disorders, which may result in obesity. You were familiarized with some of the effects autophagy can have on our body. Since this is a relatively new field of study, one has to expect that many other benefits are yet to be revealed. We may hope that the researches will continue and that in the future there will be more studies conducted on humans since that is the only way we will definitely know what happens in the human body when it has a full working process of autophagy.

What is more important for everyone reading this book is how one can easily and safely induce the process of autophagy. Here, in this book, we have discussed many types of diets and fasting as well as exercising. So, regardless of whether you are accustomed to fasting and dieting, you may find something that suits you here in this book. You will find both fasting methods that are adjustable to almost any lifestyle as well as methods that are more rigorous and stricter. These might need some sort of introduction to the fasting, like some other methods of fasting. When you get used to fasting, you can move to these more rigorous fasting methods. Practically, almost all of these methods of fasting that are presented in this book will help you activate the process of autophagy. Especially if you combine them with keto or low carb diet and exercise. This would be the jackpot of autophagy activations.

One has to bear in mind that if they have some diseases or disorders, or even if they seem healthy, they should consult their doctor, just so that they are sure that they can start any of these procedures. Also, if you feel any discomfort, if you don't feel well, you should again consult your doctor to be safe. Apart from that, I hope that you will try some of these methods of fasting or dieting, as well as exercising. You are now sure that besides those obvious health reasons, these are even more beneficial than one might think, especially under the surface.

The next step you can make is to try to adjust your lifestyle so that you can fast whenever you want to and exercise as much as you can. These two activities will help you lead a healthier life even if we don't take into account the benefits of autophagy. However, the health benefits of one such process will and must only give us a boost of motivation to endure even longer hours of fasting and exercise a couple of sets of exercise more. In the end, I hope that you understood clearly how important autophagy is for our lives and that you will try to induce it as often as possible, especially when you get older.

Thanks

I would like to thank you for taking the time to read and examine the content of this book. I hope that you benefited from this book at least in some way. If you found this information useful in any way, I would greatly appreciate the feedback.

If you can, please leave a review. Leaving a review allows me to see where I can improve and increases the chance other people will see this book which will possibly help them as well.

About the Author

______________________ is an author, anthropologist, bioengineer, specialist in human health and performance. She has 15 years of experience in conducting various studies and researches on human health and performance related topics. She has proven to be among the leading researchers in the field of bioengineering and anthropology. Currently, she is working on a new study which is closely connected to the findings in this book.

References

- Autophagy is essential to support skeletal muscle plasticity in response to endurance exercise - Scientific Figure on ResearchGate. Available from: https://www.researchgate.net/figure/Exercise-and-autophagy-in-skeletal-muscle-While-a-single-boot-of-endurance-exercise_fig3_264794740 [accessed 13 Oct, 2019]

- Beyer, M. (2019). Alternate-day fasting has health benefits for healthy people. Retrieved from https://www.medicalnewstoday.com/articles/326213.php

- Bjarnadottir, A. (2018). The Beginner's Guide to the 5:2 Diet. Retrieved from **https://www.healthline.com/nutrition/the-5-2-diet-guide#section3**

- Boya, P., Codogno, P., & Rodriguez-Muela, N. (2018). Autophagy in stem cells: repair, remodelling and metabolic reprogramming. Development **2018 145: dev146506 doi: 10.1242/dev.146506**

- Brandt, N., Gunnarsson, T. P., Bangsbo, J., & Pilegaard, H. (2018). Exercise and exercise training-induced increase in autophagy markers in human skeletal muscle. *Physiological reports*, *6*(7), e13651. doi:10.14814/phy2.13651

- Citroner, G. (2019). Alternate-Day Fasting Means Avoiding Food for 36 Hours. Is That Healthy? Retrieved from **https://www.healthline.com/health-news/is-fasting-on-alternate-days-good-for-your-health#No-diet-is-one-size-fits-all**

- Deretic, V., & Levine, B. (2018). Autophagy balances inflammation in innate immunity. Autophagy, 14(2), 243 - 251. doi:10.1080/15548627.2017.1402992

- Eenfeldt, A. (2019). A Low-carb Diet for Beginners. Retrieved from https://www.dietdoctor.com/low-carb

- English, N. (2019). Autophagy: The Real Way to Cleanse Your Body. Retrieved from https://greatist.com/live/autophagy-fasting-exercise

- Fung, J. (2017). Fasting and Autophagy. Retrieved from https://medium.com/personal-growth/fasting-and-autophagy-9f4e97596ed4

- Fung, J. (2019). Intermittent Fasting for Beginners. Retrieved from https://www.dietdoctor.com/intermittent-fasting

- *García-Prat, L., Perdiguero, E., Ortet, L., Ruiz-Bonilla, V., Gutarra, S., & Serrano, A.L. (2018). Cell autophagy, a key process in muscle regeneration during aging. Retrieved from https://www.somma.es/articles/cell-autophagy-key-process-muscle-regeneration-during-aging*

- Hale, A. N., Ledbetter, D. J., Gawriluk, T. R., & Rucker, E. B., 3rd (2013). Autophagy: regulation and role in development. Autophagy, 9(7), 951 - 972. doi:10.4161/auto.24273

- He, C., Sumpter, R., Jr, & Levine, B. (2012). Exercise induces autophagy in peripheral tissues and in the brain. *Autophagy*, *8*(10), 1548 - 1551. doi:10.4161/auto.21327

- Ives, L. (2018). Can the science of autophagy boost your health? Retrieved from https://www.bbc.com/news/health-44005092

- Jarreau, P. (2019). The 5 Stages of Intermittent Fasting. Retrieved from https://lifeapps.io/fasting/the-5-stages-of-intermittent-fasting/

- Khandia, R., Dadar, M., Munjal, A., Dhama, K., Karthik, K., Tiwari, R., Chaicumpa, W. (2019). A Comprehensive Review of Autophagy and Its Various Roles in Infectious, Non-Infectious, and Lifestyle Diseases: Current Knowledge and Prospects for Disease Prevention, Novel Drug Design, and Therapy. Cells, 8(7), 674. doi:10.3390/cells8070674

- Kubala, J. (2018). The Warrior Diet: Review and Beginner's Guide. Retrieved from https://www.healthline.com/nutrition/warrior-diet-guide

- Lahiri, V. & Klionsky, D. J. (2018). Eat Yourself to Live: Autophagy's Role in Health and Disease. Retrieved from **https://www.the-scientist.com/features/eat-yourself-to-live-autophagys-role-in-health-and-disease-30024**

- Lawton, Z. (2019). Coffee, Intermittent Fasting and Autophagy. Retrieved from **https://lifeapps.io/fasting/coffee-intermittent-fasting-and-autophagy/**

- Leonard, J. (2018). Seven ways to do intermittent fasting. Retrieved from **https://www.medicalnewstoday.com/articles/322293.php**

- Lindberg, S. (2018). Autophagy: What You Need to Know. Retrieved from **https://www.healthline.com/health/autophagy**

- Link, R. (2018). 16/8 Intermittent Fasting: A Beginner's Guide. Retrieved from **https://www.healthline.com/nutrition/16-8-intermittent-fasting#right-for-you**

- Netea-Maier, R. T., Plantinga, T. S., van de Veerdonk, F. L., Smit, J. W., & Netea, M. G. (2016). Modulation of inflammation by autophagy: Consequences for human disease. Autophagy, 12(2), 245-260. doi:10.1080/15548627.2015.1071759

- Rogers, K. (2016). Autophagy. Retrieved from https://www.britannica.com/science/autophagocytosis

- Rubinsztein, D. C., Codogno, P., & Levine, B. (2012). Autophagy modulation as a potential therapeutic target for diverse diseases. Nature reviews. Drug discovery, 11(9), 709-730. doi:10.1038/nrd3802

- Salyer, J. (2017). The Top 5 Muscular Endurance Exercises. Retrieved from https://www.healthline.com/health/fitness-exercise/muscular-endurance-exercises

- Schwalm, C., Jamart, C., Benoit, N., Naslain, D., Premont, C., Prevet, J., Van Thienen, R., Deldicque, L., & Francaux, M. (2015). Activation of autophagy in human skeletal muscle is dependent on exercise intensity and AMPK activation. *The FASEB Journal*, Vol.29, No. 8

- Shulman, S. (2019). Exactly What Happens to Your Body When You Skip a Meal, According to Dietitians. Retrieved from **https://www.prevention.com/weight-loss/a20470631/effects-of-skipping-meals/**

- Su, T.T. (2018). Cellular plasticity, caspases and autophagy; that which does not kill us, well, makes us different. Open Biology, 8-11. http://doi.org/10.1098/rsob.180157

- Wen, X., & Klionsky, D. J. (2016). Autophagy is a key factor in maintaining the regenerative capacity of muscle stem cells by promoting quiescence and preventing senescence. Autophagy, 12(4), 617 - 618. doi:10. 1080/15548627. 2016. 1158373

- Wright, J. (2018). The 24 Hour Fast: Quickest Way To Lose That Stubborn Fat? Retrieved from **https://athleticmuscle.net/24-hour-fast/**

- Yun, C. W., & Lee, S. H. (2018). The Roles of Autophagy in Cancer. International journal of molecular sciences, 19(11), 3466. doi:10. 3390/ijms19113466